4 KINDS

OF PEOPLE
THE LORD
WILL HEAL

Amb. Promise Ogbonna

Unless otherwise indicated, all Scriptural quotations are from the New King James Version

Write Amb Promise Ogbonna
Author and Publisher:
Ontop Life Publishers Company
Send Amb Promise Ogbonna a mail at: info@heavenow.org
Visit Amb. Promise Ogbonna's Website: https://www.heavenow.org
E-mail: ontoplifepublishers@gmail.com
Tel: +234 8060638053, +234 8053995257, +234 8027829586

CONTENTS

WHY I WROTE
THIS BOOK!

I am sent to Publish All the Words of God's Heavenly Kingdom Life for the Restoration of all.

I am not writing human philosophy. I am not writing as a hobby neither am I writing to entertain but to bring Spiritual light, impart, Spiritual, Wisdom and Power to build your faith and transform your life! I have a Mandate from The Lord Jesus Christ to write and these Words are published to meet man's needs in every area of life! This Book, therefore, is published in obedience to the Command of the Lord to make His Words of Life and Wisdom, Solutions and Power available to address every aspect of human needs.

I can say as Paul wrote "My message and my preaching were not in the persuasive language of philosophy, but in demonstration of the Spirit and of power; in order that your faith should rest, not on human philosophy, but on the power of God." 1Corinthians 2:4-5 (BBE)

"For the Kingdom of God is based, not on words, but on power." 1Corinthians 4:20 (BBE)

The Life Publishing Mandate

The Lord sent me to Publish All The Words of His Heavenly Kingdom Life for ALL mankind!

Jesus' last words is to Preach and Publish the Goodnews with proofs to every creature and among all nations (Mark 13:10; 16:15; Matthew 24:14).

The Lord gave us the Goodnews to publish and spread among all nations (Psalm 68:11; Mark 13:10).

In the Book of Esther, the enemy wrote and spread the words of death worldwide to destroy God's people and souls that God loves. [See Esther 3].

But at the command of the king, a new decree and words of life were written and spread to reach everyone (every creature) everywhere that the first words of death had reached. [See Esther 8].

This is our task. We have been given the New Covenant, Heavenly Kingdom, Words of Life to publish and spread to reach every creature everywhere worldwide. The Goodnews is that no one needs to die again! The old decree has been changed. Everyone can now live and enjoy peace and prosperity where each lives. That is why Ontop Mission Life Publishers Company. We are Publishing, Spreading and Bringing the Gospel of Christ and All the Words of life to every creature everywhere.

I will like to share some of the encounters with the Lord Jesus Christ that gave birth to The Life Publishing Mandate and why this Book and my other books:

1. On 2-5-95, Jesus Christ and I stood on the balcony of a great beautiful mansion in Heaven whose foundation I couldn't see (see Amos 9:6). He showed me Preachers, driven by selfishness and being used by the enemy, walking on people's heads and shoulders as their platform to preach. The people were hungry, thirsty, weeping, trampled upon and yet yearning for the TRUTH (see Amos 8:11-13). I saw My Lord shaking His head in disgust. He also brought to my view those in hell and I saw their agony and pain and what a sight it was! Afterward, as we beheld the abuse of His people, He pointed His right hand towards them and said to me, "See what is happening to the people I died for. "The Lord Jesus gave me A WELL USED COPY OF THE BIBLE and said to me "GO and tell them (The Preachers and The People) to Repent and Believe The Gospel Only and they will be Restored." I asked 'How

will I do it? And He said to me, "BE SEPARATE! Go, I send YOU as My Ambassador and Witness with My Authority and Power: Publish The Word, Stop anything after their destruction, Raise, Build and Plant them as My Ambassadors. Let them know the truth. Teach All The TRUTH and Spread them as My Seed ALL over the earth and restore all things."

2. On 6-7-96, The Lord Jesus Christ came to me again and said, "It is well" and gave me a copy of THE BIBLE and said to me, "Take: This is My Staff of Office" – My Authority and Power. After The LORD gave me His Staff of Office [The Word], I saw something like a mist or cloud appear out of the Word and as I watched, a horse emerged from 'within the mist' and jumped about and stopped. The Lord told me The Word is creative and created the horse and is My Rod for working Miracles, Wonders and Signs. I am to Go with it to all, as Moses went with his ROD, and "Stop anything after man's destruction, Bring Healing, Liberty and Restoration to all; Raise, Build and Plant Christ's Ambassadors everywhere and Restore all things."

3. On 20-5-97, I was given a BIBLE and 2 BIROS by Arch. Benson A. Idahosa in a conference that took place in a place like a stadium. And he said to me, "Go and Proclaim and Publish The Everlasting Gospel of Jesus Christ worldwide and deliver the full benefits to all. This Gospel of The Kingdom must be preached in all the world for a witness unto all nations!

4. On 18-11-03, The Lord spoke to me again ON WRITING, and said to me "Write all the hidden mysteries I show you and I will ensure it gets to all the Nations. Prophetic writings is what unveils, reveals, makes known the revelation of the mystery hidden for ages long past. The surest way of unveiling the Gospel and proclaiming Jesus Christ the Lord, is through prophetic writings as God commanded so that all nations will believe and obey God.

5. On 26-11-03, The Lord spoke to me saying, "Write what people can read and understand. It's most important. Your writing must be readable and understandable. Write in such a way that a primary school pupil can read and understand My Words. "The common people heard me gladly." Everyone must read and

understand My Words that you write.

6. On 2-10-04, The Lord Jesus explained to me the vision of 2one fifths s /95 where I Stood with Him on the Balcony of the Mansion in Heaven and He showed me Preachers using the shoulders and heads of people as their platform to preach. They were hungry, thirsty and trampled underfoot yet yearning for the reality. And The Lord commanded me to WRITE and publish His Words for the downtrodden and for all."

7. On10-12-04, The Lord said to me "Write in a book all the Words that I have spoken to you" and He gave me Jeremiah 30:2.

8. On 04-04-05, The Lord said to me "Publish the Word and bring healing, liberty and restoration to all everywhere." See Psalm 68:11 and Psalm 107:20.

9. On 23-12-05, The Lord said to me: Publish The Words, Publish The Works, Publish The Wonders, Make My Deeds Known, and Let Everyone See My Glory Everywhere.

10. On 01-03-13, The Holy Ghost said to me:
Publish the Works of Jesus Christ everywhere
Advertise the Doings of Jesus Christ the Lord.
Make known the Miracles of Jesus Christ the Lord.
Bind the Testimony of the Acts of the Lord Jesus Christ's
Be My Witness of all My Signs and Wonders everywhere.
Share Testimonies of All I AM Doing forever.
Go and Tell All everywhere of All My Miracles and Wonders and Signs and All I have done and
commanded you.

The Lord said to me "All who believe that I sent you and receive you as My Ambassador and receive your Words as My Words will experience all the Father sent me to make available to humanity!"

Like Peter, I can tell you "We have not followed cunningly devised fables, when we made known unto you the power and coming of our Lord Jesus Christ, but were eyewitnesses of his majesty." 2Peter 1:16

Beloved, every Word written in this Book is from The Lord and are His Wisdom and Heaven's Solutions packaged and released to deal with your challenges, solve your problems and meet your needs.

Read with an open heart, Believe and Receive The Truth and Pick the Lessons and engage them.

I know you will experience The One who is The Author, Perfecter and Finisher of your faith and Who is The Real Author of this Book. He is Jesus Christ, The Son of The Living God. And He is the Same yesterday and today and forever!

"O LORD, how manifold are Your works! In wisdom You have made them all. The earth is full of Your possessions." Psalm 104:24

I guarantee you that you will never be the same again as you embrace God's Wisdom in This Book!

God Bless you.

Your brother and His Steward for the benefit of all,
Ambassador Promise Ogbonna

THE HEAVENLY MANDATE & VISION

The Heavenly Mandate

To Preach The Everlasting Gospel to Everyone everywhere, Stop anything after man's destruction, Bring Healing, Liberty and Restoration to ALL; Raise, Build and Plant All as Christ's Ambassadors on His Living Mission everywhere and Restore all things!

The Heavenly Vision

To Restore All Things Everywhere at All Cost and By All Means! Acts 3:21

FIRST WORDS

4 KINDS OF PEOPLE THE LORD WILL HEAL

Every sick person that needs healing need to know how to connect with God's healing power and provision.

I want you to be sure of one thing: YOU will be healed and delivered from that evil sickness and disease that you may have presently.

On the 06-04-05 The Lord said to me "Go, Teach Healing to Infinity!" This Is Your Core Job. Teach on The Seed To Infinity! Bring Healing to the sick.

On the 7-1-12 The Lord said to me Heal a Zillion! It was also written and given to me as a Book. Proverbs 13:17 "A Trustworthy or Faithful envoy or Ambassador is health and Brings Healing."

On the 9-1-12 The Lord said to me: Your Job Description is to Bring Healing to The Sick Everywhere! Acts 10:38. He sent His Word [made flesh] and healed them and delivered them from their destructions. Ps 107:20.

On the 28-2-12 The Lord said to me: Focus on This One Thing: Focus on Healing! And Bring Healing to The Sick Everywhere. Luke 10:18-19,3-9; Acts 10:38; John 17:18

Remember The Core Job: Teach on the Seed To Infinity! Go, Teach Healing To Infinity! Heal A Zillion! Bring Healing to the sick everywhere! Heal All Oppressed by the devil. Stop Anything After Man's Destruction. Bring Healing, Liberty and Restoration to All!

On the 12-11-16, "Healing from Christ" was written and given to me: "Bring Healing from Christ to The Sick!" BRING HEALING FROM CHRIST TO THE SICK! The full price has been paid.

God says in 1Peter 2:24 "Who Himself bore our sins in His own body on the tree, that we, having died to sins, might live for right-eousness--by whose stripes you were healed."

Matthew 8:16-17 "When evening had come, they brought to Him many who were demon-possessed. And He cast out the spirits with a word, and healed all who were sick, that it might be ful-filled which was spoken by Isaiah the prophet, saying: "He Himself took our infirmities And bore our sicknesses."

Healing is available for all today. You need to understand the Four (4) Kind of people Jesus healed and Why. That is reason for this book. Read and apply and be blessed. Peace!

CHAPTER 1

*4 KINDS OF PEOPLE JESUS CHRIST
WILL HEAL AND MEET THEIR NEEDS*

Every sick person that needs healing need to know how to connect with God's healing power and provision.

I want you to be sure of one thing: YOU will be healed and delivered from that evil sickness and disease that you may have presently.

On the 06-04-05 The Lord said to me "Go, Teach Healing to Infinity!" This Is Your Core Job. Teach on The Seed To Infinity! Bring Healing to the sick. Proverbs 13:17; Psalm 107:20; Acts 10:38.

The Lord said to me to tell the Sick: "Receive My sent Ambassador, accommodate him, provide for him, hear his Word, Believe, Act on his Word and you will be healed and free from all evils." Proverbs 13:17; Luke 10:5-9

On the 24-4-05 The Lord spoke to me saying "God's Highest Secret Or Mystery Revealed Is The Seed."

My Core Job Is To Teach on "The Seed" To All. The Seed Is The Master Key To All Of God's Works - Eternal Life, Healing, Health, Prosperity and Dominion Over All. No harvest can be expected until the seed is sown. Ge 8:22. Whoever embraces The Seed System has embraced dominion. Genesis 1:26-29; 1Peter 1:23; Mark 4:3,14. Luke 8:11

On the 29-12-05 The Lord said to me "Sow The Seed and Teach

On The Seed To Infinity" Sow Is The Message! "Sow and Teach On The Seed To Infinity!" Luke 8:11

Remember the Core Job:

Go, Teach on the Seed To Infinity!

Teach Healing to Infinity!

On the 7-1-12 The Lord said to me Heal a Zillion! It was also written and given to me as a Book. Ps 107:20; Proverbs 13:17 "A Trustworthy or Faithful envoy or Ambassador is health and Brings Healing." Luke 10:5-9,19

On the 9-1-12 The Lord said to me: Your Job Description is to Bring Healing to The Sick Everywhere! Acts 10:38

On the 28-2-12 The Lord said to me: Focus on This One Thing: Focus on Healing! And Bring Healing to The Sick Everywhere. Luke 10:18-19,3-9; Acts 10:38; John 17:18

Remember The Core Job:

Teach on the Seed To Infinity!

Go, Teach Healing To Infinity!

Heal A Zillion!

Bring Healing to the sick everywhere!

Heal All Oppressed by the devil.

Stop Anything After Man's Destruction

Bring Healing, Liberty and Restoration to All!

On the 12-11-16, "Healing from Christ" was written and given to me: "Bring Healing from Christ to The Sick!" BRING HEALING FROM CHRIST TO THE SICK! The full price has been paid.

God says in 1Peter 2:24 "Who Himself bore our sins in His own body on the tree, that we, having died to sins, might live for right-eousness--by whose stripes you were healed."

Matthew 8:16-17 "When evening had come, they brought to Him many who were demon-possessed. And He cast out the spir-its with a word, and healed all who were sick, that it might be ful-filled which was spoken by Isaiah the prophet, saying: "He Himself took our infirmities And bore our sicknesses."

Notice Jesus sent me as the Father sent Him. John 17:18

Proverbs 13:17 "A faithful Ambassador is health and brings healing and health!"

Therefore, The Lord said to me: Heal a Zillion! Bring Healing to the sick everywhere!

"And into whatsoever house ye enter, first say, Peace be to this house. And if the son of peace be there, your peace shall rest upon it: if not, it shall turn to you again. And in the same house remain, eating and drinking such things as they give: for the labourer is worthy of his hire. Go not from house to house. And into whatsoever city ye enter, and they receive you, eat such things as are set before you: And heal the sick that are therein, and say unto them, The kingdom of God is come nigh unto you." Luke 10:5-9

Christ's Ambassadors Living Mission, Jesus Mission Headquarters Runs Healing Campaigns, Healing Explosions, Healing Revolutions and Holds "Healing Sessions" wherever man is found!

WHO WILL THE LORD HEAL?

(1) The Disciples

Mathew 14:22-36 "Immediately Jesus made His disciples get into the boat and go before Him to the other side, while He sent the multitudes away. And when He had sent the multitudes away, He went up on the mountain by Himself to pray. Now when evening came, He was alone there. But the boat was now in the middle of the sea, tossed by the waves, for the wind was contrary. Now in the fourth watch of the night Jesus went to them, walking on the sea. And when the disciples saw Him walking on the sea, they were troubled, saying, "It is a ghost!" And they cried out for fear. But immediately Jesus spoke to them, saying, "Be of good cheer! It is I; do not be afraid." And Peter answered Him and said, "Lord, if it is You, command me to come to You on the water." So, He said, "Come." And when Peter had come down out of the boat, he walked on the water to go to Jesus. But when he saw that the wind was boisterous, he was afraid; and beginning to sink he cried out, saying, "Lord, save me!" And immediately Jesus stretched out His hand and caught him, and said to him, "O you of little faith, why did you doubt?" And when they got into the boat, the wind ceased. Then those who were in the boat came and worshiped Him, saying, "Truly You are the Son of God." When they had crossed over, they came to the land of Gennesaret. And when the men of that place recognized Him, they sent out into all that surrounding region, brought to Him all who were sick, and begged Him that they might only touch the hem of His garment. And as many as touched it were made perfectly well.

Why did Jesus walk on water? To Reach His sent ones on The Living Mission.

He walked on water to meet and join the ones He sent on His living mission and who went in obedience to His word.

At 03.00am, when it was dark, against the fierce winds, full of fear, with fierce waves beating against their ship. Jesus came to them walking on water.

Jesus will do anything, use any means to reach and help His sent ones on The Living Mission He is sent to accomplish.

From Mathew 14:13-14,22,34-36 we see Jesus express compassion on the sick must be healed and anyone who is on his way on The Living Mission will be attacked by the enemy but will also see Jesus "walk in water" to reach him if need be

No disciple can lack healing, divine health or anything else. In Luke 22:35 "

Proofs that Jesus Healed the Disciples

i. Jesus went to Peter's house and healed the mother in law. Jesus cannot heal Peter's mother in law and leave Peter or his wife and children sick. He will gladly heal them before reaching out to his mother in law. Jesus healed everybody sick in Peter's house.

Matthew 8:14-17 says "Now when Jesus had come into Peter's house, He saw his wife's mother lying sick with a fever. So' He touched her hand, and the fever left her. And she arose and served them. When evening had come, they brought to Him many who were demon-possessed. And He cast out the spirits with a word, and healed all who were sick, that it might be fulfilled which was spoken by Isaiah the prophet, saying: "He Himself took our infirmities and bore our sicknesses."

Luke 4:38-41 "And he arose out of the synagogue, and entered into Simon's house. And Simon's wife's mother was taken with a great fever; and they besought him for her. And he stood over her, and rebuked the fever; and it left her: and immediately she arose and ministered unto them. Now when the sun was setting, all they that had any sick with divers diseases brought them unto him; and he laid his hands on every one of them, and healed them. And devils also came out of many, crying out, and saying, Thou art Christ the Son of God. And he rebuking them suffered them not to speak: for they knew that he was Christ."

ii. Jesus said it is sufficient for a disciple to be like His Master and Jesus was never sick.. but was like the Father having nothing from the devil in Him.

Luke 6:40 "The disciple is not above his master: but **every one that is perfect shall be as his master. {that...: or, shall be perfected as his master}**

John 14:9,30 "Jesus said to him, "Have I been with you so long, and yet you have not known Me, Philip? He who has seen Me has seen the Father..."the ruler of this world is coming, and he has nothing in Me."

iii. One of the disciples John the Beloved said in 1 John 1:1-7 "That which was from the beginning, which we have heard, which we have seen with our eyes, which we have looked upon, and our hands have handled, of the Word of life; (For the life was manifested, and we have seen it, and bear witness, and shew unto you that eternal life, which was with the Father, and was manifested unto us;) That which we have seen and heard declare we unto you, that ye also may have fellowship with us: and truly our fellowship is with the Father, and with his Son Jesus Christ. And these things write we unto you, that your joy may be full. This then is the message which we have heard of him, and declare unto you, that God is light, and in him is no darkness at all. If we say that we have fellowship with him, and walk in darkness, we lie, and do not the truth: But if we walk in the light, as he is in the light, we have fellowship one with another, and the blood of Jesus Christ his Son cleanses us from all sin."

Remember when he cleanses from sin, He also cleanses from ALL SICKNESSES. "He forgives all our sins and He heals all our sicknesses." Psalm 103:3]

iv. Jesus said to them in John 6:2,63 "Then a great multitude followed Him, because they saw His signs which He performed on those who were diseased...It is the Spirit who gives life; the flesh profits nothing. The words that I speak to you are spirit, and they are life."

v. Jesus asked them whether they lacked anything all the while they were with Him and running around for Him on different assignments and they said They lacked nothing. They didn't lack health. Luke 22:35 "And he said unto them, **When I sent you without purse, and scrip, and shoes, lacked ye any thing? And they said, Nothing.**"

vi. Jesus gave them power over all devils behind every sickness and disease and that power was to keep them fit to be able to meet the needs of those they were sent to and give them such as they were freely given and had received. Matthew 10:1,7,8 "And when he had called unto him his twelve disciples, **he gave them power against unclean spirits, to cast them out, and to heal all manner of sickness and all manner of disease**...And as ye go, preach, saying, The kingdom of heaven is at hand. **Heal the sick, cleanse the lepers, raise the dead, cast out devils: freely ye have received, freely give.**"

Luke 9:1-6 "Then **he called his twelve disciples together, and gave them power and authority over all devils, and to cure diseases. And he sent them to preach the kingdom of God, and to heal the sick.** And he said unto them, Take nothing for your journey, neither staves, nor scrip, neither bread, neither money; neither have two coats apiece. And whatsoever house ye enter into, there abide, and thence depart. And whosoever will not receive you, when ye go out of that city, shake off the very dust from your feet for a testimony against them. **And they departed, and went through the towns, preaching the gospel, and healing everywhere.**"

vii. Not one the Disciples of Jesus died sick. Read the story of their deaths. John the Beloved could not be killed by a hot boiling oil where he was put into with his head in the boiling oil. All the disciples possessed ETERNAL LIFE. 1John 5:11-13 "And this is the record, that God hath given to us eternal life, and this life is in his Son. He that hath the Son hath life; and he that hath not the Son of God hath not life. These things have I written unto you that believe on the name of the Son of God; that ye may know that ye have eternal life, and that ye may believe on the name of the Son of God." The Lord freed all His disciples from every sickness and disease and preserved them blameless spirit and soul and body just as he promised He will in Psalm 121:5-8 and as He did in John 10:27-30 and John 17:2-12.

"The LORD is thy keeper: the LORD is thy shade upon thy right hand. The sun shall not smite thee by day, nor the moon by night. The LORD shall preserve thee from all evil: he shall preserve thy soul. The LORD shall preserve thy going out and thy coming in from this time forth, and even for evermore." Psalm 121:5-8

""My sheep hear My voice, and I know them, and they follow Me. "And I give them eternal life, and they shall never perish; neither shall anyone snatch them out of My hand. "My Father, who has given them to Me, is greater than all; and **no one is able to snatch them out of My Father's hand. "I and My Father are one.**" John 10:27-30. Jesus and the Father had one common purpose: to keep and secure His own from the wicked. And He kept His disciples.

"As You have given Him [Jesus Your Son] authority over all flesh, that He should give eternal life to as many as You have given Him. "And this is eternal life, that they may know You, the only true God, and Jesus Christ whom You have sent. "I have glorified You on the earth. I have finished the work which You have given Me to do. "And now, O Father, glorify Me together with Yourself, with the glory which I had with You before the world was. "I have manifested Your name to the men whom You have given Me out of the world. They were Yours, You gave them to Me, and they have kept Your word. "Now they have known that all things which You have given Me are from You. "For I have given to them the words which You have given Me; and they have received them, and have known surely that I came forth from You; and they have believed that You sent Me. "I pray for them. I do not pray for the world but for those whom You have given Me, for they are Yours. "And all Mine are Yours, and Yours are Mine, and I am glorified in them. "Now I am no longer in the world, but these are in the world, and I come to You. Holy Father, keep through Your name those whom You have given Me, that they may be one as We are. "While I was with them in the world, I kept them in Your name. Those whom You gave Me I have kept; and none of them is lost except the son of perdition, that the Scripture might be fulfilled." John 17:2-12. **Notice what Jesus said: "While I was with them in the world, I kept them in Your name. Those whom You gave Me I have kept; and none of them is lost except the son of perdition, that the Scripture might be fulfilled."** Jesus lost none of His disciples to the devil or his evil demons and unclean spirits or to sickness or disease or to the storms or even evil men and killers. He kept all of them safe. Glory be to God!

And He is the same today and will heal, keep and preserve all His true disciples.

(2) The Crowd of helpless and harassed people

Matthew 15:10 Then Jesus called to the crowd to COME and HEAR. Listen", He said, and try to understand. See Luke 8:19-21 Those that heard and obeyed the words Jesus spoke He called, "My Mother, My brothers, and My sisters. Which means when anyone comes to Him, Hears the word of God and obeys it, whatever a man can do for his mother, brothers and sisters, the same will Jesus do for the person. One can be exempted from what happens to the crowd if one hears and obey The Word of God

Mathew 15:10 "When He had called the multitude to Himself, He said to them, "Hear and understand:"

Mathew 12:46-50 "While He was still talking to the multitudes, behold, His mother and brothers stood outside, seeking to speak with Him. Then one said to Him, "Look, Your mother and Your brothers are standing outside, seeking to speak with You." But He answered and said to the one who told Him, "Who is My mother and who are My brothers?" And He stretched out His hand toward His disciples and said, "Here are My mother and My brothers! "For whoever does the will of My Father in heaven is My brother and sister and mother." See Mark 3:31-35.

His disciples and everyone else that made up the crowd came to Jesus with their various needs. And He told them to hear and understand His teachings. Why? So that they will obey and do the word of God. Why? Because all who do so qualify as His NEW FAMILY and enjoy all the full benefits of God's family and household.

You can become a member of God's new family. Everyone who is a part of God's new family He will bless, heal, deliver and meet every other need such may have.

Jesus shows us that What defiles a man are his words resulting from his thoughts.

Mathew 15:10-20 says "When He had called the multitude to Himself, He said to them, "Hear and understand: "Not what goes into the mouth defiles a man; but what comes out of the mouth, this defiles a man." Then His disciples came and said to Him, "Do You know that the Pharisees were offended when they heard this saying?" But He answered and said, "Every plant which My heavenly Father has not planted will be uprooted. "Let them alone. They are blind leaders of the blind. And if the blind leads the blind, both will fall into a ditch." Then Peter answered and said to Him, "Explain this parable to us." So, Jesus said, "Are you also still without understanding? "Do you not yet understand that whatever enters the mouth goes into the stomach and is eliminated? "But those things which proceed out of the mouth come from the heart, and they defile a man. "For out of the heart proceed evil thoughts, murders, adulteries, fornications, thefts, false witness, blasphemies. "These are the things which defile a man, but to eat with unwashed hands does not defile a man."

Note: Those offended by The Living Word always will work against God's sent messengers. BUT THEY MUST BE INGNORED. (Mathew 15:12-14).

Therefore, IGNORE those who are offended by His Teaching on THE KINGDOM, GIVING, PROSPERITY, HEALING, DELIVERANCE, RESTORATION, AMBASSADORS etc.

Ignore those who get offended by The Living Word and are always to fight or work against it. Please ignore them. In Matthew

13:13-15 Jesus said whoever hears His Words and understands what He said will be healed. "Therefore speak I to them in parables: because they seeing see not; and hearing they hear not, neither do they understand. And in them is fulfilled the prophecy of Esaias, which saith, By hearing ye shall hear, and shall not understand; and seeing ye shall see, and shall not perceive: For this people's heart is waxed gross, and their ears are dull of hearing, and their eyes they have closed; lest at any time they should see with their eyes, and hear with their ears, and should understand with their heart, and should be converted, and I should heal them. Hearing the word and understanding it are His pathway or process to healing.

Proofs that Jesus Healed all The Crowd that came to hear Him.

i. Every Word of God Jesus was sent to preach was to bring Healing to the people. Psalm 107:20 "He sent his word, and healed them, and delivered them from their destructions." And Matthew 4:4:23-24 says "And Jesus went about all Galilee, teaching in their synagogues, and preaching the gospel of the kingdom, and healing all manner of sickness and all manner of disease among the people. And his fame went throughout all Syria: and they brought unto him all sick people that were taken with divers diseases and torments, and those which were possessed with devils, and those which were lunatick, and those that had the palsy; and he healed them."

ii. Every Word Jesus spoke, according to Scriptures, was health to all their flesh because they were spirit and life. Proverbs 4:20-22 "My son, attend to my words; incline thine ear unto my sayings. Let them not depart from thine eyes; keep them in the midst of thine heart. For they are life unto those that find them, and health to all their flesh." "It is the Spirit who gives life; the flesh profits nothing. The words that I speak to you are spirit, and they are life." John 6:63

iii. The people came to hear Jesus and to be healed by Him of their sicknesses and diseases for God's Power was present to heal whenever and wherever He spoke. "But so much the more went there a fame abroad of him: and great multitudes came together to hear, and to be healed by him of their infirmities...And it came to pass on a certain day, as he was teaching, that there were Pharisees and doctors of the law sitting by, which were come out of every town of Galilee, and Judaea, and Jerusalem: and the power of the Lord was present to heal them." Luke 5:15,17

iv. Jesus healed all the people that came to hear Him. Luke 6:17-19 "And he came down with them, and stood in the plain, and the company of his disciples, and a great multitude of people out of all Judaea and Jerusalem, and from the sea coast of Tyre and Sidon, which came to hear him, and to be healed of their diseases; And they that were vexed with unclean spirits: and they were healed. And the whole multitude sought to touch him: for there went virtue out of him, and healed them all."

(3) The Outcasts from the Covenant or Disqualified Sinners

Jesus healed every sinner that came to Him without an exception!

And here are the Proofs Jesus Healed Sinners.

i. Jesus healed the daughter of the woman from Tyre and Sidon.

Mathew 15:21-28 "Then Jesus went out from there and departed to the region of Tyre and Sidon. And behold, a woman of Canaan came from that region and cried out to Him, saying, "Have mercy on me, O Lord, Son of David! My daughter is severely demon-possessed." But He answered her not a word. And His disciples came and urged Him, saying, "Send her away, for she cries out after us." But He answered and said, "I was not sent except to the lost sheep of the house of Israel." Then she came and worshiped Him, saying, "Lord, help me!" But He answered and said, "It is not good to take the children's bread and throw it to the little dogs." And she said, "Yes, Lord, yet even the little dogs eat the crumbs which fall from their masters' table." Then Jesus answered and said to her, "O woman, great is your faith! Let it be to you as you desire." And her daughter was healed from that very hour."

The disqualified "Gentile" woman that Jesus called a dog and whose daughter was demon possessed and oppressed was not born again. She was a sinner; a dog! She was not included in the covenant, so, she and her daughter were unqualified and not included in God's provisions. Yet she came to Jesus as a sinner and notice what she did:

a. She pleaded or prayed for a long while asking Jesus Christ to have mercy on her and heal her daughter. But Jesus Christ didn't say a word to her. Mathew 15:21-23

b. Jesus spoke up and said to her and said "I was sent (ONLY) to help God's lost sheep the people of Israel. Yet she refused to give up and go away but continued to follow and plead for mercy.

c. Jesus ignored her for a long while yet she persisted in Faith and still came to Jesus and worshipped him.

d. After worshipping without any response from Jesus Christ, she spoke up and pleaded again for help. Notice how she Pleaded AGAIN: She said, "LORD, Help me" Mathew 15:25

e. Jesus Christ responded. "It isn't right to take food from the Children and throw it to the dogs". The woman could have gotten offended by the response she got yet she remained focused on her mission and didn't bother about the name she was called by Jesus nor the attitude and response of the disciples. Notice in verses 22-26, that she didn't bother she was called a dog, but calmly responded and said to Jesus Christ that he was true to have called her a dog and agreed as the Lord has said she was unfit to have her daughter healed by Christ. For it was not right to give dogs the food meant for the children, "but" she went on to say to Jesus that the dogs cannot be denied of the crumbs that fell from their master's table. The dogs are allowed to eat the crumbs and scraps that fall beneath their masters' table.

f. And Jesus responded and said to her "Dear woman, "Your faith is great. Your request is granted" And her daughter was instantly healed"

The unqualified, unbeliever with all her sins and exclusion from God's agenda for divine provision still got her needs met by her actions

She came to Jesus

She pleaded and prayed and was not attended to.

She was discouraged by both Jesus Christ and His Disciples.

She was excluded from the provision.

She worshiped and pleaded and prayed again.

She was told that what she asked for was not meant for her as she was not included in God's agenda and plan.

She acknowledged The Living Word and declared that she cannot be denied the crumbs as that will be enough for her needs.

She got what she wanted.

The unqualified can still get anything they want if only they can believe and stand on The Living Word no matter what they see.

ii. Mary Magdalene was a notorious sinner yet Jesus cast out seven (7) devils out of her, forgave her many sins and healed her.

"And one of the Pharisees desired him that he would eat with him. And he went into the Pharisee's house, and sat down to meat. And, behold, a woman in the city, which was a sinner, when she knew that Jesus sat at meat in the Pharisee's house, brought an alabaster box of ointment, And stood at his feet behind him weeping, and began to wash his feet with tears, and did wipe them with the hairs of her head, and kissed his feet, and anointed them with the ointment. Now when the Pharisee which had bidden him saw it, he spake within himself, saying, This man, if he were a prophet, would have known who and what manner of woman this is that touches him: for she is a sinner. And Jesus answering said unto him, Simon, I have somewhat to say unto thee. And he saith, Master, say on. There was a certain creditor which had two debtors: the one owed five hundred pence, and the other fifty. And when they had nothing to pay, he frankly forgave them both. Tell me therefore, which of them will love him most? Simon answered and said, I suppose that he, to whom he forgave most. And he said unto him, Thou hast rightly judged. And he turned to the woman, and said unto Simon, Seest thou this woman? I entered into thine house, thou gave me no water for my feet: but she hath washed my feet with tears, and wiped them with the hairs of her head. Thou gave me no kiss: but this woman since the time I came in hath not ceased to kiss my feet. My head with oil thou didst not anoint: but this woman hath anointed my feet with ointment.

Wherefore I say unto thee, Her sins, which are many, are forgiven; for she loved much: but to whom little is forgiven, the same loveth little. And he said unto her, Thy sins are forgiven. And they that sat at meat with him began to say within themselves, Who is this that forgives sins also? And he said to the woman, Thy faith hath saved thee; go in peace." Luke 7:36-50

"And it came to pass afterward, that he went throughout every city and village, preaching and shewing the glad tidings of the kingdom of God: and the twelve were with him, And certain women, which had been healed of evil spirits and infirmities, Mary called Magdalene, out of whom went seven devils, And Joanna the wife of Chuza Herod's steward, and Susanna, and many others, which ministered unto him of their substance." Luke 8:1-3

"Now when Jesus was risen early the first day of the week, he appeared first to Mary Magdalene, out of whom he had cast seven devils." Mark 16:9

iii. Jesus healed the Roman centurion's servant. He was a sinner.

"Now when he had ended all his sayings in the audience of the people, he entered into Capernaum. And a certain centurion's servant, who was dear unto him, was sick, and ready to die. And when he heard of Jesus, he sent unto him the elders of the Jews, beseeching him that he would come and heal his servant. And when they came to Jesus, they besought him instantly, saying, That he was worthy for whom he should do this: For he loveth our nation, and he hath built us a synagogue. Then Jesus went with them. And when he was now not far from the house, the centurion sent friends to him, saying unto him, Lord, trouble not thyself: for I am not worthy that thou shouldest enter under my roof: Wherefore neither thought I myself worthy to come unto thee: but say in a word, and my servant shall be healed. For I also am a man set under authority, having under me soldiers, and I say unto one, Go, and he goeth; and to another, Come, and he cometh; and to my servant, Do this, and he doeth it. When Jesus heard these things, he marveled at him, and turned him about, and said unto the people that followed him, I say unto you, I have not found so great faith, no, not in Israel. And they that were sent, returning to the house, found the servant whole that had been sick." Luke 7:1-10

iv. Jesus healed the Paralytics. Both were sinners

a. "And he entered into a ship, and passed over, and came into his own city. And, behold, they brought to him a man sick of the palsy, lying on a bed: and Jesus seeing their faith said unto the sick of the palsy; Son, be of good cheer; thy sins be forgiven thee. And, behold, certain of the scribes said within themselves, this man blasphemes. And Jesus knowing their thoughts said, wherefore think ye evil in your hearts? For whether is easier, to say, thy sins be forgiven thee; or to say, Arise, and walk? But that ye may know that the Son of man hath power on earth to forgive sins, (then saith he to the sick of the palsy,) Arise, take up thy bed, and go unto thine house. And he arose, and departed to his house." Matthew 9:1-7

b. "After this there was a feast of the Jews, and Jesus went up to Jerusalem. Now there is in Jerusalem by the Sheep Gate a pool, which is called in Hebrew, Bethesda, having five porches. In these lay a great multitude of sick people, blind, lame, paralyzed, waiting for the moving of the water. For an angel went down at a certain time into the pool and stirred up the water; then whoever stepped in first, after the stirring of the water, was made well of whatever disease he had. Now a certain man was there who had an infirmity thirty-eight years. When Jesus saw him lying there, and knew that he already had been in that condition a long time, He said to him, "Do you want to be made well?" The sick man answered Him, "Sir, I have no man to put me into the pool when the water is stirred up; but while I am coming, another steps down before me." Jesus said to him, "Rise, take up your bed and walk." And immediately the man was made well, took up his bed, and walked." John 5:1-9

(4) The Vast Crowd who came for Healing

Jesus healed the vast crowd or multitudes that followed Him.

Scriptural Proofs from Scriptures that Jesus Healed Great multitudes of sick people.

i. "Jesus departed from there, skirted the Sea of Galilee, and went up on the mountain and sat down there. Then **great multitudes came to Him**, having with them **the lame, blind, mute, maimed, and many others**; and they laid them down at Jesus' feet, and He healed them. So the multitude marveled when **they saw the mute speaking, the maimed made whole, the lame walking, and the blind seeing;** and they glorified the God of Israel. Now Jesus called His disciples to Himself and said, "I have compassion on the multitude, because they have now continued with Me three days and have nothing to eat. And I do not want to send them away hungry, lest they faint on the way." Then His disciples said to Him, "Where could we get enough bread in the wilderness to fill such a great multitude?" Jesus said to them, "How many loaves do you have?" And they said, "Seven, and a few little fish." So He commanded the multitude to sit down on the ground. And He took the seven loaves and the fish and gave thanks, broke them and gave them to His disciples; and the disciples gave to the multitude. So they all ate and were filled, and they took up seven large baskets full of the fragments that were left. Now those who ate were four thousand men, besides women and children." Mathew 15:29-38

The Vast Crowd came with their sick ones to Jesus Christ. They brought to Jesus people who were lame, blind, crippled, maimed, dumb, etcetera and He HEALED AND FED THEM ALL.

They continued with Jesus for 3 days. After the day one healing encounter, most of them could have left that first day but they did not. **They continued with Him for three days.**

Those who continue with Him will always see him rise to meet their needs.

All those who "climbed the mountain of the LORD" to be with Him will see Him rise up to meet their needs.

The Lord God says in Isaiah 2:2-3 "Now it shall come to pass in the latter days That the mountain of the LORD'S house Shall be established on the top of the mountains, And shall be exalted above the hills; And all nations shall flow to it. Many people shall come and say, "Come, and let us go up to the mountain of the LORD, To the house of the God of Jacob; He will teach us His ways, and we shall walk in His paths." For out of Zion shall go forth the law, And the word of the LORD from Jerusalem."

This Scripture is repeated in Micah 4:1-2 "Now it shall come to pass in the latter days That the mountain of the LORD'S house Shall be established on the top of the mountains, And shall be exalted above the hills; And peoples shall flow to it. Many nations shall come and say, "Come, and let us go up to the mountain of the LORD, To the house of the God of Jacob; He will teach us His ways, And we shall walk in His paths." For out of Zion the law shall go forth, And the word of the LORD from Jerusalem."

Hebrews 12:12-25 says "But you have come to Mount Zion and to the city of the living God, the heavenly Jerusalem, to an innumerable company of angels, to the general assembly and church of the firstborn who are registered in heaven, to God the Judge of all, to the spirits of just men made perfect, to Jesus the Mediator of the new covenant, and to the blood of sprinkling that speaks better things than that of Abel. See that you do not refuse Him who speaks."

What is unique about The Mountain of The Lord?

Isaiah 25:6-8 and Isaiah 33:24 makes it very clear that the Lord says "And in this mountain The LORD of hosts will make for all people A feast of choice pieces, A feast of wines on the lees, Of fat things full of marrow, Of well-refined wines on the lees. And He will destroy on this mountain The surface of the covering cast over all people, And the veil that is spread over all nations. **He will swallow up death forever, And the Lord GOD will wipe away tears from all faces;** The rebuke of His people He will take away from all the earth; For the LORD has spoken." "**And the inhabitant will not say, "I am sick";** The people who dwell in it will be forgiven their iniquity."

"Jesus departed from there, skirted the Sea of Galilee, and went up on the mountain and sat down there. Then great multitudes came to Him, having with them the lame, blind, mute, maimed, and many others; and they laid them down at Jesus' feet, and He healed them. So the multitude marveled when they saw the mute speaking, the maimed made whole, the lame walking, and the blind seeing; and they glorified the God of Israel." Mathew 15:29-31

ii. "And great multitudes followed him; and he healed them there." Matthew 19:2

iii. "And the blind and the lame came to him in the temple; and he healed them." Matthew 21:14

iv. "And in that same hour he cured many of their infirmities and plagues, and of evil spirits; and unto many that were blind he gave sight. Then Jesus answering said unto them, Go your way, and tell John what things ye have seen and heard; how that the blind see, the lame walk, the lepers are cleansed, the deaf hear, the dead are raised, to the poor the gospel is preached." Luke 7:21-22

v. "But when Jesus knew it, he withdrew himself from thence: and great multitudes followed him, and he healed them all." Matthew 12:15

vi. "And Jesus went forth, and saw a great multitude, and was moved with compassion toward them, and he healed their sick." Matthew 14:14

vii. "And Jesus went about all Galilee, teaching in their synagogues, and preaching the gospel of the kingdom, and healing all manner of sickness and all manner of disease among the people. And his fame went throughout all Syria: and they brought unto him all sick people that were taken with divers diseases and torments, and those which were possessed with devils, and those which were lunatick, and those that had the palsy; and he healed them. And there followed him great multitudes of [healed] people from Galilee, and from Decapolis, and from Jerusalem, and from Judaea, and from beyond Jordan." Matthew 4:23-25

Notice the makeup of the GREAT MULTITUDES that came to The Lord on the Mount and that followed Him everywhere He went. They include:

1. The Disciples on His Living Mission.

2. The Crowd of sinners that came to Him Hear and be healed by Him of their diseases.

3. The **Great multitudes of the sick and diseased that came to**

Him, having with them **the lame, blind, mute, maimed, etc.**

4. The Unquantified many others; that demonstrated great Faith and trust.by climbing the mountain and remaining with Him for three days in spite of the discomfort and inconvenience.

You see the above kind of people will always have Jesus meet their needs no matter where they are or their circumstances and needs.

Notice these fundamental lessons and always remember them:

1. At the darkest hour of any challenging situations, be it storms or adversity or financial crises or any other need Jesus Christ will walk on water to meet the needs of His sent ones and Ambassadors on His Living Mission. Mathew 14:22-34.

2. At the expense of his relatives, disciples and associates, Jesus Christ will meet the needs of all that hear His word and obey Him by doing whatever He says. Mathew 15:10; Luke 8:19-21.

3. At the expense of The Chosen Ones He is ONLY sent to bless, Jesus Christ will rise and meet the needs of all who demonstrate Great faith in Him. Mathew 15:21-28

4. Against every economic, social, geographical or racial biases, Jesus Christ will meet the needs of all who follow him to His Mountains or other inconvenient and uncomfortable and impossible locations and stay with Him there against all odds. Mathew 15:29-39.

Note the following:

1. Jesus will stop all negative circumstances to meet the needs of His Disciples and sent ones on The Living Mission. Mathew 14:22.

2. Jesus will ignore and by pass all the religious workers and ministers of the word to bless the Crowds that come to him, hears The Living Word and obeys it. Mathew 15:1-20; Luke 8:19-21.

3. Jesus will by-pass the covenant, chosen seed of Abraham to bless the heathen when they demonstrate great faith in His Mercy and Mission. Mathew 15:21-28.

4 Jesus will bypass all protocols and laws to heal, bless and prosper all who come to Him on the mountain and chose to CAMP

or stay with Him in spite of the odds. Mathew 15:29-37; Isaiah 2:2-4; Micah 4:1-5.

Jesus came for people! And He focused on meeting the need of the people.

In Luke 4:18-19, Jesus declared His Mission and Manifesto: "The Spirit of the Lord is upon me, because he hath anointed me to preach the gospel to the poor; he hath sent me to heal the brokenhearted, to preach deliverance to the captives, and recovering of sight to the blind, to set at liberty them that are bruised, To preach the acceptable year of the Lord."

He came for people not for projects. People were The project of the Lord Jesus Christ.

"And Jesus went about all the cities and villages, teaching in their synagogues, and preaching the gospel of the kingdom, and healing every sickness and every disease among the people. But when he saw the multitudes, he was moved with compassion on them, because they fainted, and were scattered abroad, as sheep having no shepherd. Then saith he unto his disciples, The harvest truly is plenteous, but the labourers are few; Pray ye therefore the Lord of the harvest, that he will send forth labourers into his harvest." Matthew 9:35-38

Luke 10:2 Therefore said he unto them, The harvest truly is great, but the labourers are few: pray ye therefore the Lord of the harvest, that he would send forth labourers into his harvest.

Jesus was mindful of the needs of all that came to Him and He met their needs.

He healed all them that had need of healing (Luke 9:11).

CHAPTER 2

HEAL ALL

God says "For all have sinned and come short of the glory of God," Romans 3:23

Sickness brings shame!

According to Romans 6:23 "The wages of sin is death."

And one of the major causes of death is sickness.

Psalms 103:3 says The Lord "Forgives all your iniquities [sins, transgression, offences], and heals all your diseases."

Psalms 118:25

Save now, I beseech thee, O LORD: O LORD, I beseech thee, Send Now Prosperity.

3John 2 shows that you can only prosper to the extent your soul prospers.

Your Spirit, Soul (Mind, Emotion, Will), and Body (Physically, Financially, Materially, Socially) are to prosper. You are to prosper in every area.

Understand that God is not interested in the death of a sinner. He is not willing that any should die and perish (in spite of his or her sins, transgressions and iniquities).

God is interested in the forgiveness and salvation of the sinner. He is unwilling to let or allow any sinner or sick one die because of His or her sins, iniquities, transgressions, offences, poverty or sickness.

We have sinned and ought to die. For all have sinned (Rom 3:23) and the wages of sin is disease or sickness or death (Rom 6:23).

Yet He chose to forgive all our sins and heal all our diseases. Psalms 103:3

And He want to do it Now – Psalms 118:25.

Now is the appointed time. 2 Corinthians 6:2

For He says: "In an acceptable time I have heard you, And in the day of salvation I have helped you." Behold now is the accepted time; behold, now is the day of salvation.

God will not postpone our forgiveness until tomorrow if we ask Him to forgive us today. Will He? NO! Therefore, He won't postpone our salvation or healing, deliverance, prosperity, restoration and blessing and fulfillment.

You are blessed. Be free in Jesus Name.

The LORD God is the HEALER OF ALL diseases. He Healed all diseases in the past. He is the same today, so He will Heal all diseases today.

He is the same forever. So He will heal all diseases forever.

If you are in need of healing, receive your healing right now.

Say aloud with your mouth now: By The stripes Jesus took on my behalf, I have been healed. So, I am free from every sickness and disease. Say so and never stop saying so and thanking the Lord for making it so!

CHAPTER 3

1. Healing is Salvation from Sickness.

James 5:15 says The Prayer of Faith SHALL SAVE THE SICK.

2. Healing is RESURRECTION from the bed or grave of SICKNESS.

James 5:15 The Lord shall Raise him (The Sick) up.

John 11:25 Jesus said, I am the Resurrection and the life.

The New Living Translation says "ANYONE who believes in me will live EVEN AFTER DYING."

3. Healing is Only Executed by the LORD who is the Resurrection and the life. James 5:15 John 11:25. The LORD Jesus is The Living Word made flesh. John 11:25 and John 1:14.

Exodus 15:26 Jesus is The Lord our Healer forever.

Proverbs 13:17 "A wicked messenger falls into trouble, But a faithful ambassador is health; brings healing and health."

Proverbs 4:22 "For they (God's Words) are life to those who find them, And health to all their flesh." Compare Acts 5:20; 1Jn 1:1-4

I Represent Christ now as His Ambassadors with exactly the Same life, Spirit and Anointing for the same work of Healing all am

Nd making man like Christ and God. John 6:63; John 17:18;

14:12; John 10:35; Psalms 82:6.

4. Healing is God's Expression of forgiveness of sins to sick and diseased and enslaved ones.

5. Healing Power is Released by faith through the sent ones. James 5:15.

6. Healing is Received by the sick and appropriated by faith. James 5:15.

7. Healing is executed by Acting (by faith) on the Word of God. James 5:15.

John 2:5 says Do as He commands. Do anything He says and you'll have the results you desire (compare James 5:18-20)

There is no one who will act on God's word today and fail to Get the desired Results as God has ordained no matter how terribly sick physically, emotionally, financially, socially, economically, spiritually or mentally.

8. Healing is God's tool to stop sickness, (The Sick), CAPTIVITY, POVERTY, BONDAGE, SLAVERY (Raise them up), and sins unbelief oppression (sins) James 5:15 + Acts 10:38;

Mark 5:26- She spent all she had and became poor because of excessive medical bills.

9. Total Healing is the LORD'S Ordained means of Raising you far above all evils and assaults. James 5:15; Ephesians 2:6

Raise, Build and Plant them, All the sick where nothing, no one, no evil could ever reach them. Salvation, Deliverance, Healing is for All. Be free.

CHAPTER 4

*JESUS THE HEALER SUBDUES
SICKNESS TO MAKE US LIKE HIMSELF*

"For our citizenship is in heaven, from which we also eagerly wait for the Savior (The Healer, the Redeemer, the Deliverer), The Lord Jesus Christ who will transform our lowly body that it may be conformed to His glorious body, according to the working by which He is able even to subdue all things to Himself."

Notice that the Lord raises up the sick. James 5:15.

Jesus the Lord, the Saviour, the Healer, the Redeemer, the Deliverer, the Giver, the Life, The Shepherd etc is ABLE to subdue all things.

He is able to subdue Satan, death, sin, poverty, sickness, oppression, captivity, demons, principalities, powers, rulers, might, dominion, all and everything that rise against His will, purpose, mission, God (His Father) will. See 1 Corinthians 15:22-26.

All things that have power to keep the body deformed, He is able to subdue so that our lowly body may be transformed to His glorious.

It is His plan that as Citizens of Heaven, we represent Him on Earth as His Ambassadors.

We cannot do so with a deformed, sickly body. Therefore, He must unfailingly subdue sickness, poverty, sin and Satan, etc to transform our body to conform to His body.

Halleluiah!

There is nothing He is able to subdue and which He came to subdue that will be able to keep you me in bondage. Never! Because He is ABLE and is still Doing all He came to Do. ALways remember that The Word says:

"For I am the LORD, I change not." Malachi 3:6

"Jesus Christ the same yesterday, and today, and forever." Hebrew 13:8

"And said, If thou wilt diligently hearken to the voice of the LORD thy God, and wilt do that which is right in his sight, and wilt give ear to his commandments, and keep all his statutes, I will put none of these diseases upon thee, which I have brought upon the Egyptians: for I am the LORD that heals thee." Exodus 15:26

"When the even was come, they brought unto him many that were possessed with devils: and he cast out the spirits with his word, and healed all that were sick: That it might be fulfilled which was spoken by Esaias the prophet, saying, Himself took our infirmities, and bare our sicknesses." Mathew 8:16-17.

CHAPTER 5

SICKNESS DOES NOT AFFECT ANY DEAD MAN. SO I CANNOT BE SICK!

Once a man dies, no sickness or/ disease can ever affect him. He is dead.

Galatians 2:20 – I have been crucified with Christ. Therefore, just as Christ Cannot ever be sick, I cannot be sick.

1 Corinthians 15:31 – I die daily" To die daily is to be free from sickness daily.

Therefore, No sickness or disease can ever have any hold on me any day just as it cannot have any hold over any dead man any day.

I cannot be sick any day, all the days of my life because "I have been crucified with Christ. I am a dead man in Christ. Again, it is written, "I die daily". That means everyday of my life, I am free from sin and free from sickness; Every day of my life!

Sin, Sickness and Satan lost their hold on me when I was crucified with Christ.

The law of sin and of death has no hold over me at all because the law of the Spirit of life in Christ Jesus has made me and set me free from the Law of sin, sickness, disease and of death. I have been made a free man in Christ Jesus. No Sickness or Disease can ever have a hold on Jesus Christ and therefore cannot ever be seen in me.

When a man dies the sickness or disease that killed him dies also.

Therefore, no evil disease plaguing mankind can come near me just as it cannot ever be near any dead man.

CHAPTER 6

THE HARVEST FOR YOUR HEALING IS NOW! SO, DON'T WAIT TILL TOMORROW

"The harvest is past, The summer is over, and we are not saved!" I weep for the hurt of my people; I stand amazed, silent, dumb with grief. Is there no medicine in Gilead? Is there no physician there? Why doesn't God do something? Why doesn't He help? Jeremiah 8:20-22, TLB

Jesus warned us saying "Do you not say, 'There are still four months and then comes the harvest'? Behold, I say to you, lift up your eyes and look at the fields, for they are already white for harvest! "And he who reaps receives wages, and gathers fruit for eternal life, that both he who sows and he who reaps may rejoice together. "For in this the saying is true: 'One sows and another reaps. I sent you to reap that for which you have not labored; others have labored, and you have entered into their labors." John 4:35-38

The Harvest is almost over and finished. The summer is almost over.

The Time is Up for your Salvation.

If the harvest and summer pass or end or is finished without your Salvation or healing, deliverance and restoration, don't blame anybody.

The summer is not to finish without God attending to your

need.

Now. Is the accepted time, Behold, now is the day of salvation.

God is in a hurry to save and heal you. You must not allow the devil nor do wicked people who do not care about your health and state hinder you from being saved and healed.

Listen; it is all about you, not anybody else. If you die Now or today, all those you think that love you will be the first to cry, then put your body in the mortuary, and go buy new clothes, some food stuff, drinks and celebrate your "glorious" exit through premature death and a life well spent [according to them] under Satanic captivity and sickness and disease.

Please hear me, you must make up your mind to live and fight the fight of faith to live. It's all about you, not all about anybody else. May God help you understand.

Today must not pass without your Salvation and healing:

Listen: There is "Medicine in Gilead – God's palace"

The Living Word is the Medicine.

Proverbs 4:20-22

20 My son, give attention to my words; Incline your ear to my sayings.

21 Do not let them depart from your eyes; Keep them in the midst of your heart;

22 For they are life to those who find them, And health to all their flesh.

You become incompatible even by sickness when you begin to use this medicine.

1 Peter 1:23

Having been born again, not of corruptible seed but incorruptible, through the word of God which lives and abides forever,

There is the physician. He is Jesus Christ the Lord. Exodus 15:26; Hebrews 13:18; Malachi 3:6

There is His prescription. I am sent here by Him to deliver it to you. All that will hear and do as I say will have the devil and disease leave them. This place here healed and whole irreversibly so.

God has made every provision and done everything required for you and everyone sick no matter the sickness or disease to be healed.

"If I have told you earthly things and you do not believe, how will you believe if I tell you heavenly things? No one has ascended to heaven but He who came down from heaven, that is, the Son of Man who is in heaven. **And as Moses lifted up the serpent in the wilderness, even so must the Son of Man be lifted up, that whoever believes in Him should not perish but have eternal life.** For God so loved the world that He gave His only begotten Son, that whoever believes in Him should not perish but have everlasting life. For God did not send His Son into the world to condemn the world, but that the world through Him might be saved. He who believes in Him is not condemned; but he who does not believe is condemned already, because he has not believed in the name of the only begotten Son of God. And this is the condemnation, that the light has come into the world, and men loved darkness rather than light, because their deeds were evil." John 3:12-19

"And they journeyed from mount Hor by the way of the Red sea, to compass the land of Edom: and the soul of the people was much discouraged because of the way. And the people spake against God, and against Moses, Wherefore, have ye brought us up out of Egypt to die in the wilderness? for there is no bread, neither is there any water; and our soul loathes this light bread. And the LORD sent fiery serpents among the people, and they bit the people; and much people of Israel died. Therefore, the people came to Moses, and said, We have sinned, for we have spoken against the LORD, and against thee; pray unto the LORD, that he take away the serpents from us. And Moses prayed for the people. **And the LORD said unto Moses, Make thee a fiery serpent, and set it upon a pole: and it shall come to pass, that every one that is bitten, when he looks upon it, shall live. And Moses made a serpent of brass, and put it upon a pole, and it came to pass, that if a serpent had bitten any man, when he beheld the serpent of brass, he lived."** Number 21:4-9

All you need to be healed and live free and healthy is available. God has helped you. Only accept His help and live.

"For He says: "In an acceptable time I have heard you, And in the day of salvation I have helped you." Behold, now is the accepted time; behold, now is the day of salvation." 2 Corinthians 6:2

"The LORD is thy keeper: the LORD is thy shade upon thy right hand. The sun shall not smite thee by day, nor the moon by night. The LORD shall preserve thee from all evil: he shall preserve thy soul. The LORD shall preserve thy going out and thy coming in from this time forth, and even for evermore." Psalms 121:5-8

"Look unto me, and be ye saved, all the ends of the earth: for I am God, and there is none else. I have sworn by myself, the word is gone out of my mouth in righteousness, and shall not return, That unto me every knee shall bow, every tongue shall swear." Isaiah 45:22-23

"He sent his word, and healed them, and delivered them from their destructions." Psalms 107:20

He brought them forth also with silver and gold: and there was not one feeble person among their tribes." Psalms 105:37

"Who Himself bore our sins in His own body on the tree, that we, having died to sins, might live for righteousness--by whose stripes you were healed." 1 Peter 2:24

"When evening had come, they brought to Him many who were demon-possessed. And He cast out the spirits with a word, and healed all who were sick, that it might be fulfilled which was spoken by Isaiah the prophet, saying: "He Himself took our infirmities And bore our sicknesses." Matthew 8:16-17

"Surely he hath borne our griefs, and carried our sorrows: yet we did esteem him stricken, smitten of God, and afflicted. But he was wounded for our transgressions, he was bruised for our iniquities: the chastisement of our peace was upon him; and with his stripes we are healed." Isaiah 53:4-5

Learn to look up to the Lord for your healing. The full price has been paid for you to be free from all evils, sicknesses and diseases. Lookup and live.

Take the physician's prescribed medicine as He made it available and be whole.

CHAPTER 7

ITS OVER WITH SIN, POVERTY, SICKNESS AND DEATH

"Comfort, yes, comfort My people!" Says your God. Speak comfort to Jerusalem, and cry out to her, That her warfare is ended, That her iniquity is pardoned; For she has received from the LORD'S hand Double for all her sins." Isaiah 40:1-2

The Lord wants all of mankind to be comforted.

Healing is bringing COMFORT to mankind. For nothing robs man of comfort than sickness and disease.

Galatians 6:9-10 "And let us not grow weary while doing good, for in due season we shall reap if we do not lose heart. Therefore, as we have opportunity, let us do good to all, especially to those who are of the household of faith."

Comfort, Comfort ye my people.

The Lord says "Comfort ye, comfort ye my people, saith your God. Speak ye comfortably to Jerusalem, and **cry unto her, that her warfare is accomplished, that her iniquity is pardoned:** for she hath received of the LORD'S hand double for all her sins."

If your sins are pardoned, then your sicknesses and diseases must be cleared away.

That means, there should be:

No more sad days

No more hard-labour

No more sad-labour

No more unpaid labour

My warfare and your warfare are accomplished and are ended.

My hard labour is accomplished. Your warfare is accomplished.

It's my time of favour. Its your time of favour.

"Thou shalt arise, and have mercy upon Zion: for the time to favour her, yea, the set time, is come." Psalm 102:13

Your sins are paid for yet you're kept in Bondage. Why?

1.Sin brought you into bondage.

2. If your sins are pardoned then your sicknesses are destroyed and removed. So, you were healed. And so, you are!

2. You live as a slave and labour yet the fruit of your labour goes to another [the Master] and not you. Notice that:

a. Jesus was made sin for me. 2 Corinthians 5:21

b. Jesus was made poor for me. 2 Corinthians 8:9

c. Jesus suffered for me.

d. Jesus died for us. Romans 5:8

e. Jesus was made sick for us.

"Who Himself bore our sins in His own body on the tree, that we, having died to sins, might live for righteousness--by whose stripes you were healed." 1 Peter 2:24

"When evening had come, they brought to Him many who were demon-possessed. And He cast out the spirits with a word, and healed all who were sick, that it might be fulfilled which was spoken by Isaiah the prophet, saying: "He Himself took our infirmities And bore our sicknesses." Matthew 8:16-17

"Therefore, since Christ suffered for us in the flesh, arm yourselves also with the same mind, for he who has suffered in the flesh has ceased from sin." 1Peter 4:1

Why must I go on suffering the penalty of sin?

Why must I labour and another eats?

No MORE, HENCEFORTH IN JESUS NAME.

CHAPTER 8

DISALLOW SICKNESS!

Refuse to allow Satan, sin, sickness to have anything to do with the body in which you live.

Any sensible man puts checks and balance, to keep away thieves from entering his home.

Satan is called a thief, not a robber

John 10:10

The thief does not come except to steal, and to kill, and to destroy. I have come that they may have life, and that they may have it more abundantly.

God's people are called Robbers, not thieves

Malachi 3:7-9

7 Yet from the days of your fathers You have gone away from My ordinances And have not kept them. Return to Me, and I will return to you," Says the LORD of hosts. "But you said, 'In what way shall we return?'

8 "Will a man rob God? Yet you have robbed Me! But you say, 'In what way have we robbed You?' In tithes and offerings.

9 You are cursed with a curse, For you have robbed Me, Even this whole nation.

A thief steals whenever he is giving an opportunity. See Ephesians 4:27

A robber creates his own opportunity and robs. He robs by

force from those he shouldn't have robbed people who have secured their property.

No thief steals from those who secures their property and are keeping watch over their possessions.

But a robber will break through your security to rob. That means, Satan cannot impose sickness on you without your consent.

You must allow him if he must get at you (James 4:7).

If you tell him off, he'll back off. You can stop all sickness, diseases henceforth if you want to and they will leave you. Refuse to allow sickness, disease and spirit of poverty to have anything to do with your body wherever you live.

Satan has no dominion over me.

Sin has no dominion over me.

Sickness has no dominion over me. Evil circumstances have no dominion over me.

The forces of darkness have no dominion over me.

CHAPTER 9

"**B**ehold what manner of love the Father has bestowed on us, that we should be called children of God! Therefore, the world does not know us, because it did not know Him. Beloved, now we are children of God; and it has not yet been revealed what we shall be, but we know that when He is revealed, we shall be like Him, for we shall see Him as He is." 1 John 3:1-2

We are really God's children people like God in every way and in every sense of the word. We've seen him as he really is and so we are like him in this world.

As He is, so are we in this

"Love has been perfected among us in this: that we may have boldness in the Day of Judgment; because as He is, so are we in this world." 1 John 4:17

How is Jesus in Heaven today?

Jesus is clothed with a glorified physical body, sin free body, sickness-free body, disease-free body, devils and demon-free body and super healthy.

"The redemption and glorification of the body of saved man (Christ's Ambassadors) is the end of the ways of God"

This is expressed through the Spirit saved and filled with The Living Word and God's life. Romans 6:23.

2 Corinthians 4:4 "Whose minds the god of this age has blinded, who do not believe, lest the light of the gospel of the glory of Christ, who is the image of God, should shine on them."

The Soul saved and filled with The Living Word and God's life.

"My son, attend to my words; incline thine ear unto my sayings. Let them not depart from thine eyes; keep them in the midst of thine heart. For they are life unto those that find them, and health to all their flesh." Proverb 4:20-22

The Body saved and fill with The Living Word and God's life.

"Always carrying about in the body the dying of the Lord Jesus, that the life of Jesus also may be manifested in our body. For we who live are always delivered to death for Jesus' sake, that the life of Jesus also may be manifested in our mortal flesh." 2 Corinthians 4:10-11

When the Physical body of man becomes saturated and filled and clothed with God's life via The Living Word (Romans 4:20-22). Man attends the highest glory of the Risen Saviour and Lord Jesus Christ and becomes the express image of the Living God.

Man attends the highest glory of the Risen Lord and God the Father when his flesh embodies the life and health of God via Jesus Christ The Living Word.

The sanctification and sanctity of the Spirit and soul depend on the Redemption of the body.

A corrupted body will breed a corrupted soul and will eventually breed a corrupted Spirit filled with unbelief.

Unbelief corrupts the Spirit man.

The Healing Mission

God's plan Has been to make man like Himself, Healthy as God is.

Genesis 1:26-28 "Then God said, "Let Us make man in Our image, according to Our likeness; let them have dominion over the fish of the sea, over the birds of the air, and over the cattle, over all the earth and over every creeping thing that creeps on the earth. So, God created man in His own image; in the image of God He created him; male and female He created them. Then God blessed them, and God said to them, "Be fruitful and multiply; fill the earth and subdue it; have dominion over the fish of the sea, over the birds of the air, and over every living thing that moves on the earth."

Jesus was anointed and He went about doing good and healing all tat were oppressed of the devil.

Acts 10:38 says "How God anointed Jesus of Nazareth with the Holy Spirit and with power, who went about doing good and healing all who were oppressed by the devil, for God was with Him."

"The Spirit of the Lord is upon me, because he hath anointed me to preach the gospel to the poor; he hath sent me to heal the brokenhearted, to preach deliverance to the captives, and recovering of sight to the blind, to set at liberty them that are bruised, To preach the acceptable year of the Lord." Luke 4:18-19

"Then he called his twelve disciples together, and gave them power and authority over all devils, and to cure diseases. And he sent them to preach the kingdom of God, and to heal the sick. And he said unto them, Take nothing for your journey, neither staves, nor scrip, neither bread, neither money; neither have two coats apiece. And whatsoever house ye enter into, there abide, and thence depart. And whosoever will not receive you, when ye go out of that city, shake off the very dust from your feet for a testimony against them. And they departed, and went through the towns, preaching the gospel, and healing everywhere." Luke 9:1-6

Matthew 10:1,7-8 "And when he had called unto him his twelve disciples, he gave them power against unclean spirits, to cast them out, and to heal all manner of sickness and all manner of disease. But go rather to the lost sheep of the house of Israel. And as ye go, preach, saying, The kingdom of heaven is at hand. Heal the sick, cleanse the lepers, raise the dead, cast out devils: freely ye have received, freely give." Matthew 10:1,7-8

CHAPTER 10

*THE TOUCH OF FAITH FOR
YOUR HEALING*

All who touched Him were healed!

"And when they came out of the boat, immediately the people recognized Him, ran through that whole surrounding region, and began to carry about on beds those who were sick to wherever they heard He was. Wherever He entered into villages, cities, or in the country, they laid the sick in the marketplaces, and begged Him that they might just touch the hem of His garment. And as many as touched Him were made well. Power was coming out of Him and All who touched were healed " Mark 6:54-56

"And He came down with them and stood on a level place with a crowd of His disciples and a great multitude of people from all Judea and Jerusalem, and from the seacoast of Tyre and Sidon, who came to hear Him and be healed of their diseases, as well as those who were tormented with unclean spirits. And they were healed.9 And the whole multitude sought to touch Him, for power went out from Him and healed them all." Luke 6:17-19

All who touched Him were healed

"And when the men of that place recognized Him, they sent out into all that surrounding region, brought to Him all who were sick, And begged Him that they might only touch the hem of His garment. And as many as touched it were made perfectly well.

She touched the hem of His clothe and got healed.

"Now a certain woman had a flow of blood for twelve years, and had suffered many things from many physicians. She had spent all that she had and was no better, but rather grew worse. When she heard about Jesus, she came behind Him in the crowd and touched His garment. For she said, If only I may touch His clothes, I shall be made well. Immediately the fountain of her blood was dried up, and she felt in her body that she was healed of the affliction. And Jesus, immediately knowing in Himself that power had gone out of Him, turned around in the crowd and said, "Who touched My clothes? Mark 5:25-30

Jesus was Anointed with The Holy Spirit and with power.

Acts 10:38 "How God anointed Jesus of Nazareth with the Holy Spirit and with power, who went about doing good and healing all who were oppressed by the devil, for God was with Him."

The Holy Spirit is upon me because He has Anointed me.

Luke 4:18

The Spirit of the LORD is upon Me, Because He has anointed Me To preach the gospel to the poor; He has sent Me to heal the brokenhearted, To proclaim liberty to the captives And recovery of sight to the blind, To set at liberty those who are oppressed; Jesus had the Power because He was Anointed.

He did Miracles and Signs and Wonders.

Acts 2:22

Men of Israel, hear these words: Jesus of Nazareth, a Man attested by God to you by miracles, wonders, and signs which God did through Him in your midst, as you yourselves also know.

Mathew 9:20-22

20 And suddenly, a woman who had a flow of blood for twelve years came from behind and touched the hem of His garment.

21 For she said to herself, "If only I may touch His garment, I shall be made well."

22 But Jesus turned around, and when He saw her He said, "Be of good cheer, daughter; your faith has made you well." And the woman was made well from that hour. Mark 5:24-34; Luke

8:43-48

The woman with the issue of blood for 12 years TOUCHED Jesus cloak and was instantly healed of her plaque of 12 years long standing.

By RECEIVIMG The Holy Spirit, I've Received the SAME Power that THE FATHER gave to Jesus Christ

Acts 1:5, 8

5 "for John truly baptized with water, but you shall be baptized with the Holy Spirit not many days from now."

8 "But you shall receive power when the Holy Spirit has come upon you; and you shall be witnesses to Me in Jerusalem, and in all Judea and Samaria, and to the end of the earth."

2 Corinthians 1:20-22

1 John 2:20, 27

John 20:21-23 + John 17:18 + John 14:12 Show that I can do also all Jesus did and more than He did because He has Given all He had/has and more – His Blood of the New Testament and His Name.

* The man touched Dr Oyedepo and was healed.

* The bleeding woman touched Frances Hunter and was instantly healed.

* Whoever will believe and touch me shall be healed of whatever ailment she / he has.

The Touch of faith works.

Peter's shadow healed.

Paul's handkerchief healed the sick.

1 Corinthians 2:9 –

What The World has not heard, seen or imagined will be dome by our hands in this era and season. Get ready for you have a prominent role to play in this move of God.

BECOME A CITIZEN OF HEAVEN TODAY!

Please note, if you are not yet a Citizen of Heaven, but desire to be, this is your opportunity. To be a citizen of Heaven, you must be from above. You must be born of God. You must be born again!

John 3:3-8,12-13

3 Jesus answered and said to him, "Most assuredly, I say to you, unless one is born again, he cannot see the kingdom of God."

4 Nicodemus said to Him, "How can a man be born when he is old? Can he enter a second time into his mother's womb and be born?"

5 Jesus answered, "Most assuredly, I say to you, unless one is born of water and the Spirit, he cannot enter the kingdom of God.

6 "That which is born of the flesh is flesh, and that which is born of the Spirit is spirit.

7 "Do not marvel that I said to you, 'You must be born again.'

8 "The wind blows where it wishes, and you hear the sound of it, but cannot tell where it comes from and where it goes. So is everyone who is born of the Spirit."

12 If I have told you earthly things, and ye believe not, how shall ye believe, if I tell you of heavenly things?

13 And no man hath ascended up to heaven, but he that came down from heaven, even the Son of man which is in heaven.

Jesus says "You must be born again to live and enjoy Heaven-now!" John 3:3,7

No matter your sin(s) and what you may have done, God wants you forgive and restored now!

John 3:13-18

13 "No one has ascended to heaven but He who came down from heaven, that is, the Son of Man who is in heaven.

14 "And as Moses lifted up the serpent in the wilderness, even so must the Son of Man be lifted up,

15 "that whoever believes in Him should not perish but have eternal life.

16 "For God so loved the world that He gave His only begotten Son, that whoever believes in Him should not perish but have everlasting life.

17 "For God did not send His Son into the world to condemn the world, but that the world through Him might be saved.

18 "He who believes in Him is not condemned; but he who does not believe is condemned already, because he has not believed in the name of the only begotten Son of God.

Remember God gives the power to become His son to everyone that receives Jesus as The Christ, The Son of The Living God or believe in His Name. John 1:12

Remember God Himself dwells in everyone who believes and confesses that Jesus is The Christ, The Son of The Living God. 1John 5:1, 4-5;1John 4:4,15

Remember God did not send His Son into the world to condemn the world but that through Him, the world might be saved. John 3:17

Beloved, AS the Father sent Jesus The Christ, even so has The Lord Jesus Christ sent me so that everyone who will believe and receive me as His Ambassador will be saved, healed, delivered and restored. The Lord said to me: As the Father sent Me, even so have I sent you! John 17:18; John 20:21

The Lord said to Me: Verily, verily I say to you, whoever receives you receives me, and whoever receives me receives the Father who sent me. John 13:20.

The Lord said to Me: Whoever rejects you rejects me, and whoever rejects Me rejects The Father who sent Me. Luke 10:16

The Lord said to Me: Behold I give unto you power to tread upon serpents and scorpions and over all the power of the enemy and nothing shall by any means hurt you. Luke 10:19

The Lord said to Me: Behold, I send in the midst of many peoples, like dew from the LORD, like showers on the grass, that tarry for no man nor wait for the sons of men. Behold, you shall be among the Gentiles, In the midst of many peoples, like a lion among the beasts of the forest, like a young lion among flocks of sheep, Who, if he passes through, both treads down and tears in pieces, and none can deliver. Your hand shall be lifted against your adversaries, and all your enemies shall be cut off. Micah 5:7-9

The Lord said to Me: You will be like the dew to all My people and creation; You shall grow like the lily, and lengthen Your roots like Lebanon. Your branches shall spread; Your beauty shall be like an olive tree, And Your fragrance like Lebanon. Those who dwell under Your shadow shall return; They shall be revived like grain, and grow like a vine. Their scent shall be like the wine of Lebanon. Hosea 14:5-7

Beloved, there is no justifiable reason under Heaven why you should ever go through ANYTHING that is not in Heaven now!

Beloved there is no justifiable reason why you should not have NOW the best God has fully paid for and credited to your personal account!

Hear Me: All things are ready. And all things are yours! What are you still waiting for? All you need to do is to believe that Jesus is the Christ, The Son of The Living God. And He sent Me to bring this Goodnews to you.

Your struggles can come to an end today. You can be enrolled into Heaven's citizenship right now. You can begin a new life today and enjoy all that is available in Heaven from this day forward. The Lord Jesus Christ who sent me confirms with undeniable proof that He is ALIVE today in the lives of those who hear my words and believes in Him [The Lord Jesus Christ] who sent me.

Jesus is alive today and the only way to prove it is for Him to do what He did before in your life today. He sent me and will prove to you that this is not a made-up story written to impress you, but His ordained will made available to make you are created to be!

The choice is yours! Rise and take what belong to you and enter your rest!

Peace now and always in Jesus Almighty Name!

Amen!!!

If You are not certain that You are Born Again as you are certain of your name, or You were once saved but went astray again, living and doing as you pleased, then say this Prayer aloud now for you to become a citizen of Heaven:

PRAYER FOR SALVATION AND RESTORATION TO HEAVEN'S CITIZENSHIP!

Dear Heavenly Father, I return to you by Faith. I am sorry for my sins. I believe in my heart that Jesus is The Christ and that He died for my sins and rose from the dead on the third day, according to Scripture, for my justification. I confess that Jesus Christ is LORD and I accept Him now as my Saviour. I believe my sins are wiped away.

I call upon The Name of The LORD for my total Healing, Liberty and Restoration.

I ask for the Gift of Your Holy Spirit, Power and Grace to follow and serve You from this day forward. And I Thank You Abba Father for doing far beyond all I have asked and can ever imagine in Jesus Name. Amen!

I Now Declare That I Am A Child of God Forever! There's no going back.

Now that you have become a Citizen of Heaven, you need to upgrade by signing up to serve as an Ambassador for Christ. That is where your security and relevance lie. There is no job in this world that can be compared to serving as The Ambassador of The King of kings and Lord of lords. The benefits are amazing. You cannot do a better or more honourable job.

You can Enlist now and become a Partner or a Member of

our Totally Empowered Ambassadors on Mission (TEAM) and see what Our Risen Lord and King Jesus Christ will transform your life into and do in, for and through you from this day as you believe and obey His Word!

I can't wait to hear from you because I believe you have been blessed and helped immensely reading this Book as much as I am writing it! I am praying for you.

ABOUT THE AUTHOR

Amb. Promise Ogbonna

Amb Promise Ogbonna is the President of Christ's Ambassadors Living Mission International Inc. aka Jesus Mission Headquarters, an all-encompassing network of ministries with a mandate focus to Preach The Everlasting Gospel to all, Stop anything after man's destruction, Bring Healing, Liberty and Restoration to all, Make ALL Christ's Ambassadors and Make Heaven-Now a Reality for All.

He is the Publisher of ONTOP Life Publishers Company with a commission to Publish the Everlasting Gospel and Bring God's Wisdom-solutions for every problem and need of mankind.

He represents The Lord Jesus Christ and serves Him as His Ambassador!

He is married and blessed with children.

OTHER BOOKS BY AMB PROMISE OGBONNA

1. The Nothingness of Satan
2. You Can Make a Fresh Start and Rule Your World
3. Restoring The Forgotten Dignity of Woman
4. Christ's Ambassadors: Re-Emergence of Rulers in
5. Why Prophet Elisha Died Sick and how to Avoid it
6. You Can Choose When to Die
7. You Shall Live and Not Die
8. Why Christians Die Sick
9. 7 Keys to Undeniable Healing
10. 8 Decisive Hours That Will Take You To The Topmost
11. Activating God's Medicine For Your Healing
12. God Cannot Fail To Heal You
13. Healing Is Your Legal Right
14. God's Final Solution to The Problem of The Black Race
15. Understanding God's Secret to Winning Life's Battles
16. 100 Years Is Minimum
17. How to Raise The Dead
18. Manifesting ss Signs and Wonders: Unlocking The Unstoppable You Regardless of Where You are Now!
19. 40 Pitfalls to Avoid in Life – Mastering The Art of Living Successfully.
20. Wisdom Seeds to Greatness In Life – Inspiring Seed-Thoughts on Being Your Best
21. God's Medicine for Incurable Diseases
22. Ambassador Promise: Jesus Christ's Official Ambassador and T. L. Osborn's Successor on Earth Today! Appearance and En-

counters with The Lord Jesus Christ, Mantles of Notable Servants of God Received and The 9 Mandates.

UPCOMING BOOKS BY AMB PROMISE OGBONNA

1. Enforcing Kingdom Wealth Transfer
2. God's Final Word on Tithes, Tithing and Offerings
3. Creating Heaven Out of Your Ruined World
4. How to Attract God's Blessing on Your Business and Career
5. How to Make Your Faith Work
6. God's Master Key to Your Dominion
7. Wisdom Keys To God's Recovery Plan
8. Jesus Christ's Teaching on Provoking Our Covenant Heritage of Prosperity
9. Why People Fail in Life –Secrets to Success without Stress

Please visit your favorite eBook retailer to discover other books by Amb Promise Ogbonna.

CONNECT WITH AMB PROMISE OGBONNA

I appreciate you reading my book. Here are my links and Social Coordinates

Send Amb Promise Ogbonna a mail at:

Visit Amb. Promise Ogbonna's Website:

Subscribe to Amb Promise Ogbonna's videos at:

Follow Amb Promise Ogbonna on Twitter:

Friend Amb Promise Ogbonna on Facebook:

Connect with Amb Promise Ogbonna on LinkedIn:

Read Amb Promise Ogbonna's Story at Wattpad:

Subscribe to Amb Promise Ogbonna's Blog at:

Follow Amb Promise Ogbonna on Instagram:

Subscribe to Amb. Promise Ogbonna's HEAVENow You Tube Channel:

Read Amb Promise Ogbonna's Smashwords Interview at

Read Amb Promise Ogbonna's Author Profile at Smashwords:

Follow Amb Promise Ogbonna at Amazon:

Connect with Amb Promise Ogbonna on Pinterest:

Read Amb. Promise Ogbonna books at Okada Books:

Get Access to all the Books of Amb Promise Ogbonna at Books2Read Universal Book Link:

JOIN AMB. PROMISE OGBONNA IN HIS HEAVENOW SERVICES

Worship with Ambassador Promise in Christ's Ambassadors Heaven-Now Services at:
Christ's Ambassadors Living Mission International [Jesus Mission Headquarters]
24 Independence Street, Behind O'Mark Schools by O'Mark Bus Stop, LASU Road, Igando Lagos
Wednesdays: 12:00-1:00pm. Hour of EmPowerment for All [Online]
Saturdays: 8:00-9:00am. Hour of Healing for All
Sundays: 8:00-9:00am. Hour of Liberty and Restoration for All
Sundays: 9:00-10:00am. Hour of Kingdom Wealth Transfer for All
Last Friday Night Monthly: 10pm. Night of Restorations for All
Ambassadors International Bible Institute: Runs Online and Offline Courses to Make Christ's Ambassadors and Make Heaven Now a reality for all. Enroll today!
HEAVENow...Making Heaven now a Reality for ALL!

OUR HEALING PRODUCTS

We are on a Mission to Bring Healing to the sick no matter their sicknesses or diseases and Restore Health, Wealth and Peace to ALL! Here are some of our Products and Services we run to Bring Healing to the sick worldwide!

1. All-Purpose Divine Healing Medicine
2. Healing Messages – Podcasts, CD, MP3 and DVD
3. Healing Books
4. Healing Leaves Magazine
5. Healing Anointing Oil
6. Healing Mantles and Clothes
7. Healing Materials
8. Healing Elixir for incurable diseases
9. Healing Songs
10. Healing Homes
11. Health Centers
12. Healing Balm

Call us today for all of your Healing needs! We are here to SERVE YOU!

OUR SPECIAL SERVICES

We Offer the following services to Churches, Ministries, Corporate Bodies, Businesses, Communities, Groups, International Bodies, NGO's, Governments, States and Nations.

1. Healing Seminars
2. Healing School
3. Healing Teams
4. Healing Outreaches and Explosions
5. World Healing Conferences
6. Health and Wealth Trainings
7. Heaven-Now Campaigns
8. Kingdom Wealth Transfer Seminars
9. God's FASTEST Prosperity Recovery Seminars
10. Heaven's Business School
11. Time and Stress Management Training
12. Leadership Responsibility Development Training

Our Services are geared towards making every person fit spirit, soul and body so that they can be empowered to deliver results competently, effectively and efficiently.

For Bookings Contact us today!

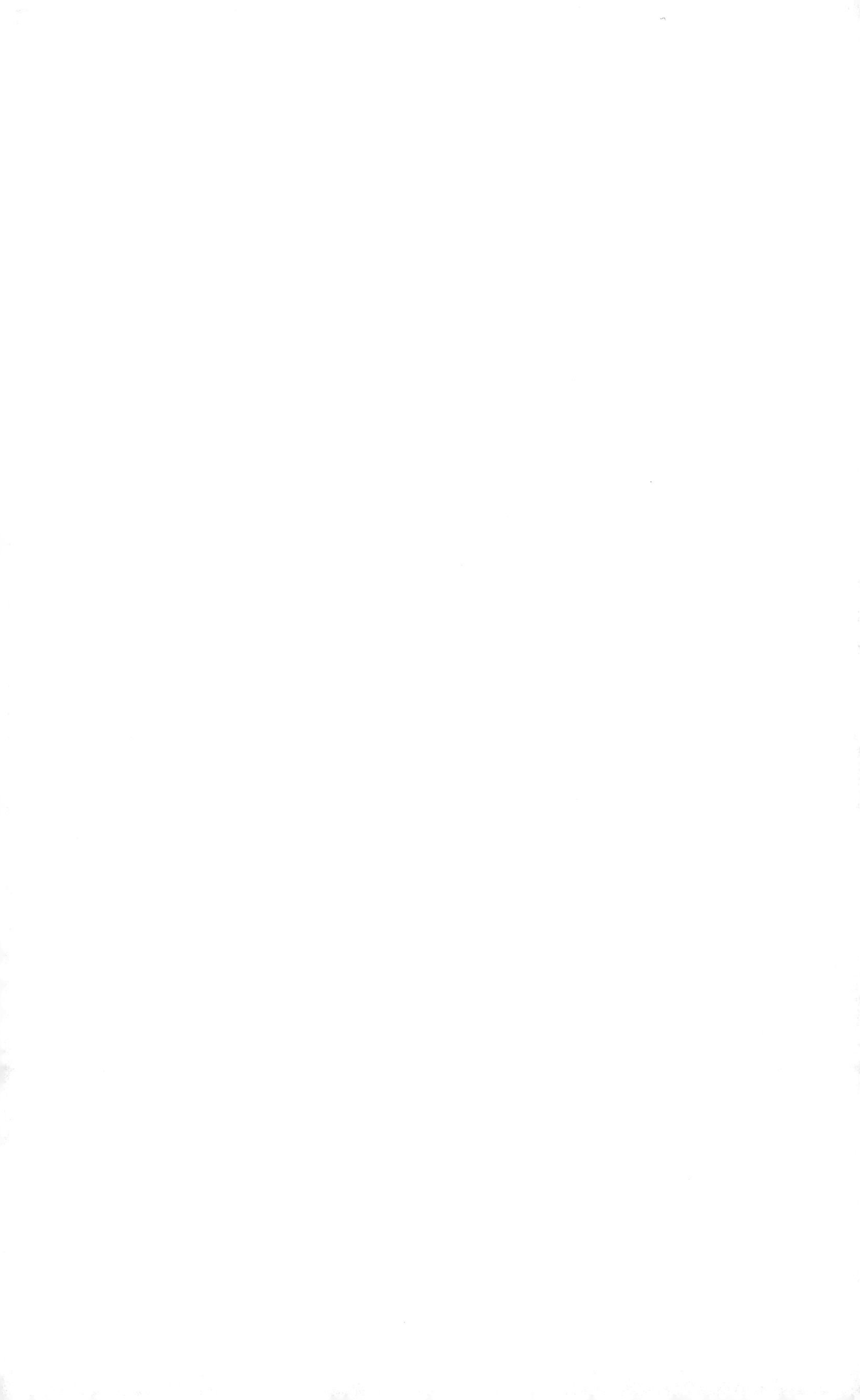